Navigating the Waves
A Dad's Guide to Coping with Mom's Mood Swings During Pregnancy

By Greig Borthwick

DEDICATION

To the mother of our future children. I will listen to you, reason with you, love you, and nurture you. We are in this together. You're the strongest person I know.

CONTENTS

Acknowledgments   i

1 The Emotional Rollercoaster   3

2 Communication is Key   21

3 Self-Care for Dads   39

4 The Role of Hormones   57

5 Preparing for Baby   67

6 Coping Strategies   89

7 Navigating Challenges   97

8 Bonding with Baby   103

9 Building a Support System   111

10 Celebrating the Journey   119

ACKNOWLEDGMENTS

Moms-to-be around the world....

We know you love us; we will support you every day. Please be nice to us, this we pray.

Chapter 1

The Emotional Rollercoaster

Understanding Hormonal Changes

During pregnancy, a woman's body under-goes significant hormonal fluctuations. These hormonal changes play a substantial role in causing mood swings. Here's an overview of some of the key hormones involved.

Estrogen:

Estrogen plays a significant role in mood and emotions during pregnancy. Here's a bit more detail on how estrogen can influence emotional fluctuations.

Neurotransmitter Impact: Estrogen can impact the production and function of neurotransmitters in the brain, including serotonin and dopamine. These neurotransmitters are closely linked to mood regulation. Changes in estrogen levels can disrupt the delicate balance of these neurotransmitters, potentially contributing to mood swings.

Emotional Sensitivity: Increased estrogen levels can make pregnant women more emotionally sensitive. What might have been a minor issue before pregnancy could now evoke a stronger emotional response. Understanding this heightened emotional sensitivity is important for partners, as it helps in providing the necessary support and empathy.

First Trimester Surges: Estrogen levels rise most significantly during the first trimester, and this is when many women experience pronounced mood swings. The combination of rapidly changing hormones and the body adjusting to pregnancy can lead to emotional fluctuations.

Progesterone:

Calming Effect: Progesterone is often referred to as the "calming hormone" because it has a relaxing effect on the body. It helps maintain the uterine lining and prevents contractions that could potentially lead to a miscarriage. This calming effect can be beneficial during pregnancy, but it's essential to note that it can interact with other hormonal changes.

Mood Swings: While progesterone's calming effect is generally beneficial, when combined with other hormonal fluctuations, it can sometimes lead to mood swings or increased emotional sensitivity. These mood swings might result from the dynamic interplay between progesterone and hormones like estrogen and hCG.

Emotional Sensitivity: The increased levels of progesterone can make a pregnant woman more emotionally sensitive. She might react more strongly to various stimuli or situations than she would outside of pregnancy. It's important for partners to recognize this emotional sensitivity and provide understanding and support.

Human Chorionic Gonadotropin (hCG):

Pregnancy Test Marker: Human Chorionic Gonadotropin (hCG) is the hormone responsible for the positive result in pregnancy tests. It's produced by the developing placenta shortly after a fertilized egg attaches to the uterine lining. Detecting hCG in a woman's urine or blood is a reliable way to confirm pregnancy.

Corpus Luteum Maintenance: One of hCG's primary roles in early pregnancy is to maintain the corpus luteum, a temporary endocrine structure in the ovaries. The corpus luteum produces progesterone, which is vital for sustaining the uterine lining and supporting the early stages of pregnancy until the placenta takes over this function. Without hCG, the corpus luteum would degenerate, leading to a drop in progesterone levels, which could jeopardize the pregnancy.

Emotional Fluctuations: Elevated hCG levels in early pregnancy can contribute to emotional fluctuations. This hormonal surge can affect mood and may be linked to symptoms like morning sickness and increased emotional sensitivity. These symptoms are often more pronounced during the first trimester when hCG levels are at their peak.

Support and Understanding: It's important for expectant fathers to be aware of the role of hCG in pregnancy and its potential influence on mood swings and other symptoms. Providing emotional support and understanding during this time can be particularly valuable, especially as the body adjusts to the surge in hCG and the many changes it brings.

Cortisol:

Stress Response: Cortisol is a hormone released by the body in response to stress. It's part of the body's natural "fight or flight" response and plays a crucial role in managing stress. During pregnancy, the body may still respond to stressors by releasing cortisol.

Mood Swings: Elevated cortisol levels, whether due to external stressors or other factors, can contribute to mood swings. When a person experiences chronic stress or heightened stress levels during pregnancy, it can lead to increased emotional reactivity and irritability. This is why managing stress is essential.

Managing Stress: Stress management is crucial during pregnancy. Expectant mothers should be encouraged to practice relaxation techniques, engage in physical activity, and seek support when needed. Partners can play a vital role in helping to reduce stress by providing emotional support, helping with daily tasks, and creating a calm and supportive environment.

Communication: Open communication about stress and its potential impact on mood swings is key. Both partners should feel comfortable discussing their feelings and concerns. Encouraging your partner to express their emotions and being an active listener can help reduce stress levels.

Understanding the relationship between cortisol, stress, and mood swings is vital for both expectant mothers and fathers-to-be. By actively managing stress and providing emotional support, couples can navigate the challenges of pregnancy more smoothly and enjoy this transformative journey together.

Oxytocin:

The "Love Hormone": Oxytocin is often referred to as the "love hormone" or "cuddle hormone" because it plays a central role in bonding, social interactions, and fostering positive emotions. This hormone is particularly vital for the formation of emotional bonds between partners, parents and children, and individuals in close relationships.

Mother-Child Bonding: During pregnancy, oxytocin is released in response to various events and stimuli, including physical touch, affection, and labor contractions. This hormone is a key player in establishing and strengthening the emotional bond between the mother and her unborn child, as well as after birth during breastfeeding and nurturing.

Emotional Sensitivity: While oxytocin promotes positive emotions and bonding, it can also make a woman more emotionally sensitive during pregnancy. Expectant mothers may experience heightened emotions, both positive and negative. This emotional sensitivity can contribute to mood swings, as everyday stressors and interactions may evoke stronger emotional responses.

Support and Understanding: It's important for partners to understand the role of oxytocin and its potential effects. Being aware of the emotional sensitivity that oxytocin can bring about can help expectant fathers provide the support, comfort, and understanding that their partners need during pregnancy.

Common Mood Swing Triggers

Understanding the hormonal changes is crucial, but it's also essential to recognize common triggers for mood swings during pregnancy. These triggers can vary from woman to woman, but some are universally common.

Hormonal Fluctuations:

Normalizing Hormonal Changes: It's essential for both partners to recognize that hormonal fluctuations are a natural and necessary part of pregnancy. These changes are not something your partner can control, and they are crucial for the healthy development of the baby and the changes occurring in her body.

Empathy and Understanding: Understanding that your partner may experience emotional ups and downs due to these hormonal fluctuations is the first step in providing support. Being empathetic, patient, and non-judgmental when your partner is going through mood swings can make a significant difference in her emotional well-being.

Effective Communication: Open and honest communication is key. Both partners should feel comfortable discussing their emotions, concerns, and needs. This allows for a deeper connection and ensures that both individuals are on the same page regarding the challenges of pregnancy.

Self-Care: Encourage your partner to engage in self-care activities that can help manage mood swings, such as relaxation techniques, exercise, and adequate rest. You, as a dad-to-be, should also practice self-care to maintain your own emotional well-being and be better prepared to support your partner.

Professional Help: In some cases, mood swings can become severe or persistent, indicating the need for professional assistance. If your partner's mood swings are causing significant distress, consider seeking guidance from a healthcare provider or mental health professional.

Fatigue:

Increased Tiredness: Pregnancy can bring about significant physical changes, such as increased blood volume and metabolic demands. These changes can lead to fatigue, especially in the first and third trimesters. Your partner may find herself feeling more tired and needing more rest than usual.

Disrupted Sleep Patterns: Pregnant women often experience disrupted sleep patterns due to physical discomfort, frequent urination, and hormonal fluctuations. These disturbances can lead to poor-quality sleep, which can exacerbate feelings of tiredness and irritability.

Mood Swings and Irritability: When someone is fatigued, they are more likely to experience mood swings and become irritable. Your partner may find it challenging to manage her emotions when she's exhausted. This can lead to mood swings and may affect her overall emotional well-being.

Offering Support: Understanding the impact of fatigue on your partner's mood is crucial. Providing support by taking on additional household tasks, encouraging her to rest, and being understanding when she needs to take breaks can be immensely helpful.

Self-Care: Encourage your partner to prioritize self-care, including napping, relaxation exercises, and maintaining a healthy diet, to combat fatigue. You can also engage in self-care
practices to ensure you have the energy and patience to support her.

Effective Communication: Encourage open communication about how fatigue is affecting her and how you can assist. Discuss strategies to manage fatigue and its impact on mood swings together.

Fatigue is a common and challenging aspect of pregnancy, and understanding its connection to mood swings can help you provide the support and care your partner needs during this period.

Physical Discomfort:

Morning Sickness: Morning sickness, characterized by nausea and sometimes vomiting, is a common pregnancy symptom, especially during the first trimester. Dealing with morning sickness can be physically and emotionally taxing. Your partner's discomfort may lead to frustration or irritability.

Backaches: The growing uterus can place additional pressure on the lower back, leading to backaches. Hormonal changes and the relaxation of ligaments can also contribute to back pain. Constant discomfort in this area can certainly lead to irritability.

Frequent Urination: The increased blood flow to the pelvic area and the growing uterus can lead to frequent urination. This can disrupt sleep, daily routines, and even lead to frustration.

Swelling and Discomfort: Swelling of the feet and ankles, as well as general physical discomfort, is not uncommon during pregnancy. This can affect mobility and comfort, leading to mood swings.

Support and Understanding: Recognizing the physical discomfort your partner may be experiencing and acknowledging the challenges it poses is essential. Providing support, helping with tasks, and offering understanding can go a long way in helping her cope.

Encourage Self-Care: Encourage your partner to engage in self-care practices that can help alleviate physical discomfort. These may include prenatal yoga, massages, and warm baths, among others.

Communication: Encourage open communication about the physical discomfort she's experiencing. Ask how you can help and be a listening ear for her concerns.

Anxiety and Worry:

Health of the Baby: Pregnancy often comes with natural worries about the health and well-being of the developing baby. Concerns can arise about prenatal tests, fetal development, and potential complications. These worries can lead to mood swings and emotional ups and downs.

The Birthing Process: Anxiety about the birthing process is entirely normal. The uncertainty surrounding labor and delivery can be a source of stress for expectant mothers. Fears of pain, complications, and the unknown can contribute to mood swings.

Becoming a Parent: The prospect of becoming a parent can be both exciting and daunting. Expectant parents may worry about their ability to care for a child, the impact on their relationship, and the changes parenthood will bring to their lives. These concerns can trigger mood swings.

Coping with Anxiety: It's crucial to address anxiety and worry during pregnancy. Encourage open communication with your partner about her fears and concerns.

Consider attending prenatal classes or seeking professional guidance to alleviate anxiety and build confidence.

Supportive Role: As a partner, offering emotional support and reassurance is invaluable. Listening to your partner's worries without judgment, being empathetic, and actively participating in the pregnancy journey can help ease her anxieties.

Education: Learning about the pregnancy process, birthing options, and parenting can help both partners feel more prepared and reduce anxiety. Knowing what to expect can provide a sense of control and confidence.

Body Image Issues:

Body Changes: Pregnancy brings about significant physical changes, including weight gain, a growing belly, breast changes, and stretch marks. These changes can make some women feel self-conscious and challenge their body image.

Self-Esteem: Struggling with body image issues can impact a woman's self-esteem and overall mood. The perception of not meeting societal beauty standards or feeling less attractive can lead to emotional distress and mood swings.

Open and Supportive Communication: Encourage open and supportive communication with your partner. Let her know that you find her beautiful and attractive, and that her body changes are a natural and vital part of the pregnancy process.

Compliments and Encouragement: Offer compliments and words of encouragement to boost her self-esteem. Remind her that her body is doing an incredible thing by growing a new life, and that these changes are a testament to her strength and resilience.

Healthy Body Image: Promote a healthy body image by emphasizing the importance of self-care, rather than achieving a specific appearance. Encourage self-acceptance and remind your partner that her body is adapting for a beautiful purpose.

Self-Care and Body Positivity: Encourage self-care practices that make your partner feel good about herself, whether it's gentle exercise, prenatal massages, or simply taking time for relaxation and self-appreciation.

External Stressors:

Work-related Stress: The demands of a job, especially when combined with pregnancy-related fatigue and discomfort, can lead to stress. Balancing work responsibilities with pregnancy can be challenging, and stress at work can contribute to mood swings.

Financial Concerns: Financial worries are common for many expectant parents. Preparing for the costs associated with pregnancy, childbirth, and the needs of a newborn can be stressful. These concerns can affect mood and well-being.

Family Issues: Family dynamics can sometimes be a source of stress during pregnancy. This can include issues with extended family, conflicts, or adjustments to changing roles and responsibilities. Such family-related stressors can impact mood swings.

Communication and Support: Effective communication and support are key in addressing these external stressors. Discuss your concerns with your partner, and actively listen to hers. Offering emotional support and working together to find solutions can help reduce stress.

Time Management: Managing time efficiently can help reduce stress related to work and personal life. This may involve setting priorities, setting boundaries at work, and delegating tasks when possible.

Seeking Professional Help: If external stressors are overwhelming and causing persistent mood swings, consider seeking the assistance of a mental health professional. They can provide strategies to manage stress and emotional well-being.

Relationship Changes:

Changing Roles and Responsibilities: Pregnancy often leads to shifts in roles and responsibilities within a relationship. Expectant mothers may experience physical discomfort and fatigue, which can affect their ability to perform certain tasks. This can sometimes lead to stress and emotional fluctuations.

Communication Challenges: Couples may experience communication challenges as they adjust to the changes brought about by pregnancy. Misunderstandings or unspoken expectations can create emotional stress and lead to mood swings.

Emotional Changes: Pregnancy can bring about emotional changes in both partners. Hormonal fluctuations in expectant mothers and the anticipation of parenthood can trigger mood swings and stress.

Support and Understanding: Open and honest communication is crucial during this time. Partners should talk about their feelings, expectations, and concerns. Offering emotional support, understanding, and patience can help couples navigate the changes and challenges of pregnancy.

Quality Time: Make an effort to spend quality time together and nurture your relationship. This can include date nights, emotional check-ins, or simply taking time to connect and bond as a couple.

Seeking Professional Help: If relationship-related stress and mood swings become overwhelming, consider seeking couples' counseling or therapy. A professional can provide guidance and strategies to improve communication and navigate relationship changes.

Understanding these triggers and the hormonal changes at play can help you empathize with your partner and provide the support and understanding she needs during this emotional rollercoaster of pregnancy.

Chapter 2

Communication is Key

Effective communication is essential for navigating the challenges and emotional fluctuations of pregnancy. This chapter explores ways to communicate effectively and provides guidance on listening and empathizing.

Effective Ways to Talk

Active Listening:

Giving Full Attention: When your partner wants to talk, make a conscious effort to give her your full attention. This means putting aside distractions, like your phone or the TV, and focusing solely on her.

Maintaining Eye Contact: Eye contact is a powerful non-verbal way to show that you're engaged in the conversation. It signals that you're actively listening and interested in what she has to say.

Avoid Interrupting: Avoid interrupting her while she's speaking. Let her finish her thoughts before you respond. Interruptions can make your partner feel unheard and can be frustrating.

Non-Verbal Cues: Use non-verbal cues like nodding or other gestures to show that you're actively listening. These cues can convey empathy and understanding.

Reflective Listening: Repeat back what your partner has said to ensure you've understood correctly. For example, you can say, "I hear you saying that you're feeling anxious about the upcoming doctor's appointment. Is that right?"

Ask Open-Ended Questions: Encourage further conversation by asking open-ended questions. These questions can prompt your partner to share more about her thoughts and feelings.

Empathetic Responses: Respond to her with empathy and understanding. Show that you, acknowledge her emotions and that you care about how she's feeling.

Active listening is a powerful tool for building trust, fostering open communication, and demonstrating your support for your partner during the emotional journey of pregnancy. It can help her feel heard, valued, and comforted during challenging times.

Use "I" Statements:

Using "I" statements is a valuable communication technique, especially when discussing concerns or feelings, as it promotes effective and non-confrontational communication. Here's a more in-depth explanation.

Expressing Emotions: "I" statements allow you to express your emotions and thoughts from a personal perspective. Instead of blaming or accusing, you focus on your own feelings, which can lead to a more constructive conversation.

Taking Responsibility: By saying, "I feel worried when..." you take responsibility for your emotions and how you react to situations. It's a way of owning your feelings and avoiding placing blame on your partner.

Non-Confrontational: "I" statements are non-confrontational and less likely to provoke defensiveness in the other person. This can lead to a more open and less emotionally charged conversation.

Encouraging Empathy: When you use "I" statements, it can encourage your partner to empathize with your feelings. It helps them understand how their actions or words affect you personally.

Effective Problem-Solving: This form of communication is effective for problem-solving because it promotes a collaborative approach. It encourages both partners to work together to find solutions rather than becoming defensive or argumentative.

Here's an example of how you can use "I" statements during pregnancy: Instead of saying, "You make me worry when you don't answer my calls," you can say, "I feel worried when I can't reach you because I care about your safety and well-being."

Using "I" statements in your communication can foster a healthier, more understanding, and supportive environment during the emotional journey of pregnancy. It's a valuable skill for addressing concerns and emotions in a constructive way.

Stay Calm:

Staying calm during discussions, especially when your partner is emotional, is an essential component of effective communication and support during pregnancy. Here's a more detailed look at the importance of remaining composed.

Emotional Support: When your partner is experiencing heightened emotions, it's important for at least one of you to remain calm. Your emotional stability can provide a supportive anchor for her during moments of stress or anxiety.

Active Listening: Staying calm allows you to engage in active listening, which involves fully understanding and empathizing with your partner's emotions. It's challenging to do this when you're emotionally charged.

Problem Solving: Calm discussions are more conducive to problem-solving. Emotional outbursts can hinder productive conversations, while composure promotes the ability to address issues and concerns effectively.

Conflict Resolution: In the event of disagreements or conflicts, maintaining your composure can prevent arguments from escalating. It sets a positive example and encourages a healthier resolution process.

Emotional Contagion: Emotions can be contagious. If you react with heightened emotions when your partner is already emotional, it can exacerbate the situation. Conversely, your calm demeanor can help soothe her emotions.

Reassurance: Remaining calm reassures your partner that you are a stable and dependable presence in her life. It can alleviate some of her stress and help her feel more secure.

While it's okay to express your feelings and concerns, doing so in a composed and respectful manner can create a more supportive and understanding atmosphere during pregnancy. Your ability to remain calm during discussions can make a significant difference in your partner's emotional well-being.

Choose the Right Time:

Selecting the right time for discussions, especially those involving important matters, is indeed crucial for effective communication and mutual understanding. Here's a more detailed look at the significance of timing:

Relaxed Atmosphere: A relaxed atmosphere encourages a more productive and open conversation. Choose a time when both you and your partner are free from immediate stressors or distractions.

Avoid Rushing: Rushed discussions can lead to miscommunication and increased tension. Try to avoid having important conversations when you or your partner are in a hurry or preoccupied with other responsibilities.

Consider Energy Levels: Pay attention to both of your energy levels. Conversations may be more productive when you're both adequately rested and not fatigued from a long day.

Emotional Readiness: Ensure that you and your partner are emotionally prepared for the conversation. Sometimes, it's beneficial to ask, "Is this a good time to talk about something important?" This shows consideration for each other's emotional state.

Minimize Distractions: Choose a setting that minimizes distractions. Silence or put away electronic devices and find a quiet space where you can focus on the conversation without interruptions.

Set Aside Quality Time: Dedicate quality time for discussions that matter. This can involve setting a specific time to sit down and talk without feeling rushed or interrupted.

Selecting the right time for conversations is a simple yet effective way to improve communication and ensure that both you and your partner are in a receptive and focused state of mind. It can lead to more productive and mutually beneficial discussions.

Be Patient:

Patience is a virtue, and it's particularly important during pregnancy when emotions can fluctuate. Here's a closer look at the significance of patience.

Emotional Rollercoaster: Pregnancy often involves a rollercoaster of emotions due to hormonal changes, physical discomfort, and the anticipation of parenthood. Recognize that mood swings and emotional fluctuations are a normal part of this journey.

Understanding Her Needs: Be attentive to your partner's needs and emotions. Sometimes, she may need time and space to process her feelings or simply have a moment to herself. Your patience allows her to do so without feeling rushed or pressured.

Non-Judgmental Support: Offer non-judgmental support and reassurance. Your patience can create a safe space where your partner feels comfortable sharing her emotions without fear of criticism.

Active Listening: Actively listen to your partner when she wants to talk. Your patience in listening, even when the conversation is emotionally charged, can make her feel heard and valued.

Respect Boundaries: Respect your partner's boundaries. If she expresses a need for space or time to herself, honor that request. It's an act of love and consideration.

Remain Steady: Your patience and emotional steadiness can help balance out the emotional fluctuations of pregnancy. It's a valuable contribution to the stability of your relationship during this transformative time.

By practicing patience and offering your partner understanding and support, you can both navigate the challenges and emotional ups and downs of pregnancy in a more harmonious and loving way.

Listening and Empathizing

Empathize:

Empathy is a powerful tool for building a strong and supportive relationship during pregnancy.

Understanding Her Perspective: Empathy involves understanding your partner's perspective, emotions, and feelings. Try to see things from her point of view, especially when she's going through emotional challenges.

Validation of Emotions: When you empathize, you validate your partner's emotions. You acknowledge that what she's feeling is real and important, even if you don't fully understand it.

Feeling Supported: Empathy can make your partner feel supported and less alone in her experience. It shows that you're there for her, that you care about her well-being, and that you're willing to share in her emotional journey.

Improved Communication: Empathy can enhance communication. When your partner feels understood and valued, she's more likely to open up and share her thoughts and feelings with you.

Reducing Emotional Distance: It bridges emotional gaps and reduces emotional distance in the relationship. Empathy fosters emotional connection and intimacy.

Shared Journey: Pregnancy is a shared journey, and empathy helps both partners experience it together. It's an opportunity for you to strengthen your bond and support each other through the challenges and joys of this transformative time.

Practicing empathy not only benefits your partner but also strengthens your relationship. It's a key component of providing emotional support during pregnancy and building a foundation of trust and understanding.

Avoid Judging:

Avoiding judgment and refraining from passing judgment on your partner's feelings and experiences is a fundamental aspect of providing emotional support during pregnancy. Here's why it's important:

Emotional Validity: Every individual's emotional experiences are valid, even if they seem irrational or unexplainable. Avoiding judgment reinforces the idea that her feelings are real and worthy of consideration.

Respect for Individual Emotions: Pregnancy can bring about a wide range of emotions, and they may not always align with logic or reason. It's important to respect your partner's emotions as a part of her unique experience.

Open Communication: Avoiding judgment encourages open and honest communication. When your partner feels that her emotions are accepted without judgment, she's more likely to
share her thoughts and feelings, which can "lead to a deeper emotional connection.

Comfort and Safety: Providing a non-judgmental space where your partner can express herself promotes her comfort and safety. She'll feel more at ease discussing her emotions and concerns without the fear of criticism.

Conflict Resolution: When you avoid judgment, it's easier to resolve conflicts and disagreements. You can discuss issues without placing blame or passing judgment, which can lead to more productive conversations.

Strengthening the Relationship: Avoiding judgment fosters trust and respect in the relationship. It strengthens the emotional bond between you and your partner and creates a more supportive and understanding environment.

In the context of pregnancy, where emotions can be heightened and unpredictable, avoiding judgment is a powerful way to provide the emotional support and empathy your partner needs during this transformative journey.

Validate Feelings:

Validation of your partner's feelings is a compassionate and effective way to provide emotional support during pregnancy.

Acknowledging Emotions: When you validate your partner's feelings, you're acknowledging that what she's experiencing is real and important. This helps her feel heard and understood.

Emotional Safety: Validation creates a safe space for your partner to express her emotions without fear of judgment or criticism. It encourages open and honest communication.

Normalization: Validating feelings helps normalize the emotional fluctuations that often come with pregnancy. It reassures your partner that her emotions are a typical and expected part of this transformative experience.

Stress Reduction: Validation can reduce stress and anxiety. When someone's feelings are validated, it can help alleviate emotional distress and create a sense of relief.

Improved Mood: Feeling validated can improve your partner's mood and emotional well-being. It can be comforting and reassuring to know that her feelings are acknowledged and accepted.

Strengthening the Relationship: Validating feelings strengthens the emotional bond between you and your partner. It demonstrates your empathy and support, fostering a more secure and connected relationship.

Remember that sometimes all a person needs to feel better is to have their feelings validated. It's a simple yet powerful way to provide emotional support and show that you care about your partner's well-being during pregnancy.

Reassure and Comfort:

Reassuring and comforting your partner during challenging moments is a crucial part of providing emotional support during pregnancy.

Emotional Security: Reassurance and comfort provide emotional security to your partner. Knowing that you're there for her and that you care can be incredibly comforting during stressful times.

Validation of Emotions: Offering reassurance acknowledges your partner's emotions and lets her know that her feelings are valid. It reinforces the idea that her experiences and concerns matter to you.

Stress Reduction: Reassurance can reduce stress and anxiety. Knowing she has your support and that you're a source of comfort can ease her emotional distress.

Strengthening Connection: It strengthens the emotional connection between you and your partner. Reassurance and comfort create a sense of unity and trust in the relationship.

Encouraging Openness: When your partner feels reassured and comforted, she's more likely to open up and share her thoughts and feelings. This can lead to more productive and supportive conversations.

Showing Care and Love: Reassurance and comfort are tangible ways of demonstrating your care and love for your partner. It's a reminder that you're in this journey together, and you're there for her.

In moments of emotional difficulty or stress during pregnancy, offering reassurance and comfort is a powerful way to show your support and love. It helps your partner feel less alone and more secure in the relationship. Effective communication, active listening, and empathy are essential tools for maintaining a healthy and supportive relationship during pregnancy. By practicing these skills, you can build a stronger connection and better navigate the emotional journey together.

Chapter 3

Self-Care for Dads

Balancing Your Needs with Mom's and Managing Stress and Anxiety.

Self-care is not just important for expectant mothers but also for dads-to-be. This chapter discusses how to balance your needs with those of the mom-to-be and provides guidance on managing stress and anxiety during pregnancy.

Balancing Your Needs with Mom's

Open Communication:

Open communication is a cornerstone of a healthy and supportive relationship during pregnancy. Here's a more detailed exploration of the importance of maintaining open communication with your partner:

Honesty: Be honest about your feelings and needs. Open communication means sharing your thoughts, concerns, and emotions in a straightforward and sincere manner.

Listening: In addition to expressing yourself, actively listen to your partner. Her perspective and concerns are equally important, and listening demonstrates your support and understanding.

Mutual Support: Open communication allows both partners to provide support to each other. By sharing your needs and concerns, you create an environment where you can be there for each other in a more meaningful way.

Conflict Resolution: When disagreements or conflicts arise, open communication is the key to resolving them constructively. It allows you to address issues and work together to find solutions.

Strengthening the Relationship: Sharing your thoughts and feelings, as well as listening to your partner, fosters a deeper emotional connection and trust in the relationship. It can help you both feel more secure and supported.

Problem Solving: Effective problem-solving is often rooted in open communication. Discussing challenges, concerns, and needs is the first step in finding solutions and making decisions together.

Open communication is a vital tool for navigating the emotional ups and downs of pregnancy and for building a strong, supportive, and understanding partnership as you prepare for parenthood. It encourages mutual respect, empathy, and love.

Support Her Self-Care:

Supporting your partner's self-care during pregnancy is not only a loving gesture but also a vital aspect of ensuring her well-being and the health of the baby. Here's why it's essential:

Maternal Health: Self-care plays a crucial role in maintaining your partner's physical and emotional health during pregnancy. This directly impacts the health and well-being of the baby.

Stress Reduction: Self-care helps reduce stress, which can have adverse effects on both the mother and the developing fetus. Encouraging self-care activities can alleviate stress and promote a healthier pregnancy.

Emotional Well-Being: Pregnancy can be emotionally challenging, and self-care routines that address emotional needs can improve your partner's mood and overall well-being.

Bonding and Connection: Engaging in self-care together, when appropriate, can be an opportunity to bond and connect as a couple. It reinforces your support and shared experiences.

Mutual Well-Being: Promoting your partner's self-care not only benefits her but also contributes to the well-being of the entire family. A healthier, happier mom is better equipped to care for the baby and nurture the family.

Respect for Autonomy: Recognizing and respecting your partner's self-care needs also demonstrates respect for her autonomy. It shows that you trust her judgment and choices.

Encourage and support your partner's self-care routines by actively participating when appropriate, respecting her needs and choices, and expressing your understanding of the importance of self-care during pregnancy. It's a way to show your love and care for both your partner and your growing family.

Find Common Ground:

Finding common ground in self-care activities is a wonderful way to strengthen your bond as a couple and prioritize your well-being during pregnancy. Here's why it's important:

Strengthening the Relationship: Engaging in shared self-care activities can strengthen your emotional connection as a couple. It's an opportunity to spend quality time together and create positive memories.

Supporting Each Other: It allows you to support each other's well-being. By participating in self-care activities together, you demonstrate your commitment to each other's health and happiness.

Creating a Positive Environment: Shared self-care can create a positive and supportive environment in your home. It fosters an atmosphere of care, understanding, and relaxation.

Stress Reduction: Many self-care activities, such as relaxation techniques or physical exercise, can help reduce stress for both partners. This contributes to a harmonious and stress-free home environment.

Preparing for Parenthood: Participating in activities like prenatal classes as a couple can help you both prepare for parenthood. It's an opportunity to learn and grow together as you anticipate the arrival of your baby.

Mutual Well-Being: Finding common ground in self-care ensures that both partners are actively involved in maintaining their well-being. It's a mutual investment in a healthy and balanced relationship.

Whether it's going for walks, attending prenatal classes, or practicing relaxation techniques together, shared self-care activities can be a source of joy, connection, and wellness for both partners during the transformative journey of pregnancy.

Delegate Responsibilities:

Delegating responsibilities and sharing household tasks is a practical and effective way to maintain balance and reduce feelings of overwhelm during pregnancy. Here's why it's essential:

Balanced Workload: Sharing household responsibilities ensures that neither partner is burdened with an unfair workload. This balance can reduce stress and prevent burnout.

Self-Care Opportunities: By sharing tasks and managing your time efficiently, you can create opportunities for both partners to engage in self-care activities. This is crucial for maintaining your emotional well-being.

Mutual Support: Delegating tasks and supporting each other in daily responsibilities fosters a sense of teamwork and mutual support. It reinforces the idea that you're in this journey together.

Quality Time: With a balanced workload, you'll have more quality time to spend together as a couple, which can enhance your emotional connection and provide opportunities for self-care.

Stress Reduction: Reducing stress and feelings of being overwhelmed is important for the health and happiness of both partners. A shared approach to household tasks can contribute to a calmer home environment.

Effective Time Management: Effective delegation and time management can help you make the most of your time, ensuring that both of you have the opportunity to engage in self-care and relaxation.

Discussing how to share the workload, delegating responsibilities, and actively supporting each other in managing household tasks is a practical way to create a more balanced and harmonious environment during pregnancy. It ensures that both partners have the time and space to focus on self-care and well-being.

Managing Stress and Anxiety

Identify Stressors:

Identifying and recognizing the stressors in your life is a vital step in managing stress and ensuring your well-being during pregnancy.

Awareness: Identifying stressors allows you to be aware of the specific challenges that may be affecting your well-being. This awareness is the first step in addressing these stressors.

Emotional Health: Stressors can have a significant impact on your emotional health. By recognizing them, you can take proactive steps to mitigate their effects and maintain your emotional well-being.

Relationships: External stressors can sometimes affect your relationships, including your relationship with your partner. Being aware of these stressors enables you to manage them and reduce their impact on your relationships.

Problem-Solving: Identifying stressors is crucial for effective problem-solving. It allows you to address the root causes of stress and find strategies to manage or alleviate them.

Self-Care: Knowing your stressors helps you prioritize self-care activities that specifically address the sources of stress in your life. This can be a proactive approach to stress management.

Stress Reduction: Recognizing stressors and addressing them can lead to a reduction in overall stress levels, contributing to your overall well-being and health.

By identifying and acknowledging stressors in your life, you can take steps to manage them and prioritize self-care during pregnancy. It's an important aspect of ensuring that you're emotionally and mentally prepared for the journey ahead.

Effective Coping Strategies:

Developing effective coping strategies for managing stress and anxiety is crucial for maintaining your well-being during pregnancy.

Stress Reduction: Effective coping strategies can help reduce stress and anxiety, which can be especially important during pregnancy when emotions may be heightened.

Emotional Well-Being: Coping strategies can improve your emotional well-being and resilience, making it easier to handle the challenges and uncertainties of pregnancy.

Health Benefits: Reducing stress and anxiety has physical health benefits as well, as chronic stress can lead to various health issues. Coping strategies can help protect your health.

Supporting Your Partner: When you're equipped with effective coping strategies, you're in a better position to provide emotional support to your partner, which is essential during pregnancy.

Modeling Behavior: Demonstrating healthy coping strategies sets a positive example for your partner and, in the future, for your child. It's an opportunity to model how to manage stress and anxiety.

Preparation for Parenthood: Developing coping strategies can prepare you for the emotional demands of parenthood. It's a valuable skill to have as you navigate the challenges and joys of raising a child.

Coping strategies can include relaxation techniques, physical exercise, mindfulness practices, and seeking professional guidance when needed. Choose strategies that work best for you and incorporate them into your self-care routine to manage stress and anxiety effectively.

Support Network:

Relying on your support network is a valuable way to manage stress and anxiety during pregnancy. Here's why your support network is essential:

Emotional Outlet: Friends, family, and support groups provide a safe space to share your feelings and experiences. Expressing yourself can be therapeutic and relieve emotional tension.

Validation: Talking to others who are or have been in similar situations can validate your feelings and experiences. It shows that you're not alone in what you're going through.

Different Perspectives: Your support network can offer different perspectives and insights that you might not have considered. This can help you approach challenges from new angles.

Shared Experiences: Expectant fathers in support groups or friends who have been through pregnancy can share their experiences, advice, and coping strategies. Learning from others can be immensely beneficial.

Social Connection: Interacting with your support network provides social connections that are essential for your emotional well-being. Loneliness and isolation can exacerbate stress and anxiety, so staying connected is important.

Practical Help: Friends and family can also offer practical help, such as assisting with household tasks, providing transportation, or even lending a listening ear when needed.

By leaning on your support network and sharing your experiences, you can better manage stress and anxiety during pregnancy. It's a reminder that you have people who care about your well-being and are there to support you through this transformative journey.

Quality Time:

Spending quality time with your partner is not only a way to strengthen your emotional connection but also an effective strategy for reducing stress and anxiety during pregnancy.

Emotional Connection: Quality time allows you to nurture and strengthen your emotional connection with your partner. It's a reminder of the bond you share and can provide a sense of security during emotional challenges.

Communication: During quality time together, you can engage in open and meaningful communication. Discussing your thoughts, concerns, and joys can help alleviate stress and anxiety by sharing the emotional load.

Shared Support: When you spend quality time together, you can provide mutual support. This support can be emotionally comforting and reassuring, helping both of you cope with stress.

Distraction and Relaxation: Quality time can serve as a distraction from stressors and a source of relaxation. Engaging in enjoyable activities together can provide a much-needed break from daily worries.

Reduced Isolation: Quality time reduces feelings of isolation and loneliness, which can contribute to stress and anxiety. It reminds you both that you're not alone on this journey.

Strengthened Relationship: Consistently spending quality time together can strengthen your relationship, making it more resilient to the challenges of pregnancy and parenthood.

Self-Care Routine:

Establishing a self-care routine that caters to your physical and emotional needs is essential for maintaining your well-being during pregnancy.

Stress Reduction: A self-care routine that includes relaxation techniques, exercise, or mindfulness practices can help reduce stress, which is crucial during pregnancy when emotions can be heightened.

Emotional Well-Being: Prioritizing self-care activities that address your emotional needs can improve your mood and overall emotional well-being. It's an important aspect of self-preservation.

Physical Health: A self-care routine may include activities like exercise or maintaining a balanced diet, which are essential for your physical health during this transformative time.

Time for Yourself: Self-care routines provide you with dedicated time for yourself. This time is crucial for relaxation, recharging, and finding a sense of balance.

Enhanced Coping: Engaging in self-care activities enhances your ability to cope with the emotional and practical challenges of pregnancy and impending parenthood.

Modeling Behavior: As an expectant father, modeling a self-care routine sets a positive example for your partner and, in the future, for your child. It teaches the importance of self-care and emotional well-being.

Your self-care routine can be tailored to your preferences and needs. Whether it involves exercise, relaxation, meditation, or other self-care activities, it's an investment in your emotional and physical well-being, which benefits both you and your family during this journey.

Professional Help:

Seeking professional assistance when stress and anxiety become overwhelming is a responsible and effective way to manage your mental and emotional well-being during pregnancy.

Specialized Guidance: Mental health professionals have the expertise to provide specialized guidance and coping strategies tailored to your unique needs and circumstances.

Stress Reduction: Professional assistance can help you effectively manage and reduce stress and anxiety, which is crucial for your own well-being and the well-being of your family.

Prevent Escalation: Addressing stress and anxiety promptly can prevent these issues from escalating into more serious mental health concerns. Early intervention is valuable.

Validation and Support: Speaking with a mental health professional can provide you with validation and emotional support. It's an opportunity to express your feelings and experiences in a non-judgmental and confidential setting.

Family Well-Being: By seeking help, you're actively taking steps to ensure your well-being, which directly impacts your ability to support your partner and your family during pregnancy and beyond.

Coping Strategies: A mental health professional can equip you with effective coping strategies and tools to navigate the emotional challenges of pregnancy and parenthood.

Don't hesitate to reach out for professional help if you feel overwhelmed by stress and anxiety. It's a courageous and proactive step that can make a significant positive impact on your mental and emotional health. Your well-being is essential, and seeking help is a sign of strength and self-care. Balancing your needs with those of the mom-to-be and effectively managing stress and anxiety is essential for your well-being and for providing the best support to your partner during this transformative time.

Chapter 4

The Role of Hormones

Understanding What's Happening Inside Mom's Body and How Hormones Affect Mood.

In this chapter, we'll delve into the physiological changes occurring within an expectant mother's body, with a particular focus on the role of hormones and their impact on mood. Understanding this aspect is key to providing support and empathy during pregnancy.

What's Happening Inside Mom's Body

Growth and Development:

Fetal growth and development is an awe-inspiring journey that spans from conception to birth. Understanding the various stages and milestones of this process can deepen your appreciation for the miracle of life and help you support your partner during her pregnancy. Here's an overview.

Conception:
- Fertilization: The journey begins when a sperm fertilizes an egg, forming a single cell called a zygote.
- Rapid Cell Division: The zygote undergoes rapid cell division, becoming a blastocyst.

First Trimester (Week 1 to Week 12):
- Organ Formation: The embryo's major organs, such as the heart, brain, and limbs, begin to form.
- Heartbeat: The baby's heart starts beating around the end of the third week.
- Placenta Development: The placenta, a vital organ for nourishing the baby, takes shape.
- Limb Buds: Tiny limb buds emerge, which will develop into arms and legs.
- End of First Trimester: By the end of the first trimester, the embryo is referred to as a fetus.

Second Trimester (Week 13 to Week 27):
- Growth Spurt: The fetus experiences a significant growth spurt, with visible features and movement.

- Senses: Senses like hearing and taste begin to develop.
- Quickening: The mother may feel the baby's movements for the first time.
- Vernix and Lanugo: The fetus is covered with vernix, a waxy substance, and lanugo, fine hair.
- Viability: The baby reaches the point of potential viability outside the womb, though still requiring intensive care.

Third Trimester (Week 28 to Birth):
- Brain Development: The brain continues to develop, and the baby gains more body fat.
- Practice Breathing: The baby practices breathing movements.
- Fetal Position: The baby usually settles into a head-down position in preparation for birth.
- Weight Gain: Rapid weight gain occurs, and the baby's movements may become more noticeable.
- Full-Term: At 37 weeks, the baby is considered full-term and ready for birth.

Birth:
- Labor: The mother experiences contractions and goes into labor, leading to the birth of the baby.

- Apgar Score: Apgar scores are used to assess the baby's overall health immediately after birth.
- Bonding: The bonding process between parents and the baby begins as they hold and care for their newborn.

Understanding the stages of fetal growth and development can help you appreciate the marvel of pregnancy and parenthood. It's a reminder that the journey you and your partner are embarking on is an incredible and life-changing experience.

Organ Systems:

Understanding how the baby's organ systems develop and function during pregnancy is a fascinating aspect of the journey to parenthood. Here's an overview of the major organ systems and their development:

Cardiovascular System:
- **Development**: The cardiovascular system begins to develop early in pregnancy. The heart starts beating around the third week, and the circulatory system takes shape.
- **Function**: The baby's heart pumps blood, which carries oxygen and nutrients from the

placenta to nourish the growing fetus. This system also helps remove waste products.

-

Respiratory System:

- **Development**: The development of the respiratory system begins during the embryonic stage and continues throughout pregnancy.
- **Function**: While the baby's lungs are not fully functional until birth, they play a crucial role in oxygen exchange. In utero, oxygen primarily comes from the mother through the placenta.

Digestive System:

- **Development**: The digestive system starts developing in the first trimester, with the formation of the mouth, esophagus, stomach, and intestines.
- **Function**: The baby's digestive system allows for the absorption of nutrients from the amniotic fluid and, later, from breast milk or formula after birth.

Nervous System:

- **Development**: The nervous system's development begins early in pregnancy, with the formation of the neural tube.

- **Function**: The nervous system includes the brain and spinal cord, which control essential functions. While the baby's brain continues to develop after birth, the nervous system is responsible for regulating vital processes like breathing and heartbeat in utero.

Each of these organ systems undergoes significant development during pregnancy to support the growing fetus. It's a testament to the remarkable process of fetal growth and the complex orchestration of different systems that ultimately result in a healthy, fully functional newborn. Understanding these developments can deepen your appreciation for the incredible journey of pregnancy and the importance of maternal health in supporting fetal development.

Placenta and Umbilical Cord:

The placenta and umbilical cord are vital structures that play essential roles in nourishing and protecting the developing baby throughout pregnancy. Here's an overview of their functions and importance:

Placenta:

- **Development**: The placenta begins forming shortly after conception and is fully developed by the end of the first trimester.

- **Functions**:

  1. **Nutrient Exchange**: The placenta acts as a bridge between the mother's and the baby's circulatory systems. It allows for the exchange of nutrients and oxygen from the mother's blood to the baby's, and the transfer of waste products from the baby's blood to the mother's for elimination.

  2. **Hormone Production**: The placenta produces hormones, such as human chorionic gonadotropin (hCG), which helps maintain the pregnancy, and human placental lactogen (hPL), which supports milk production in the mother's breasts.

  3. **Protection**: It acts as a protective barrier, preventing harmful substances, such as some bacteria and viruses, from reaching the baby.

  4. **Waste Removal**: The placenta also serves as a waste disposal system, removing waste products produced by the baby.

Umbilical Cord:

- **Development**: The umbilical cord connects the baby to the placenta and begins forming around the fifth week of pregnancy.
- **Functions**:
  1. **Transportation**: The umbilical cord serves as a lifeline, transporting oxygen and nutrients from the placenta to the baby and carrying waste products, like carbon dioxide, away from the baby to be eliminated by the mother's body.
  2. **Protection**: It contains a special substance called Wharton's jelly, which provides protection against compression and ensures the cord's blood vessels remain functional.
  3. **Communication**: The umbilical cord plays a role in the communication between the baby and the mother's body, allowing for the regulation of fetal growth and development.

The placenta and umbilical cord are marvels of nature, providing a nurturing and protective environment for the developing baby. They ensure that the baby receives the essential nutrients and oxygen required for growth while helping to safeguard against potential harm. Understanding their roles highlights the intricacies of the pregnancy journey and the importance of maternal health and well-being in supporting fetal development.

Significant hormonal changes occur in an expectant mother's body during pregnancy, which we covered in chapter 1. Understand the roles of estrogen, progesterone, hCG, cortisol, and oxytocin. All of these hormones are intensified throughout each trimester. These fluctuations can lead to mood swings and emotional ups and downs. Gain insight into these mood swings to help calm your partner during challenging moments.

Chapter 5

Preparing for Baby

Getting the Nursery Ready and Attending Prenatal Classes.

In this chapter, we'll explore two essential aspects of preparing for the arrival of your baby: getting the nursery ready and attending prenatal classes. These preparations are integral to ensuring that your home is welcoming and safe for your newborn and that both you and your partner are well-informed and ready to face the challenges and joys of parenthood.

Getting the Nursery Ready

Nursery Essentials:

Setting up a nursery is an exciting and essential part of preparing for your baby's arrival. To ensure a safe and comfortable nursery, here's a list of nursery essentials:

1. **Crib**: A safe and sturdy crib is the most critical item. Look for one that meets current safety

standards and has no drop sides. Make sure to use a firm mattress and fitted crib sheets.

2. **Changing Table**: A changing table with ample storage space for diapers, wipes, and baby clothes can make diaper changes more convenient.

3. **Rocking Chair or Glider**: A comfortable chair for feeding and soothing your baby is a must. Consider one with padded cushions and armrests.

4. **Dresser**: A dresser provides storage for baby clothes and essentials. It can double as a changing table if you place a changing pad on top.

5. **Baby Monitor**: A baby monitor allows you to keep an eye (and ear) on your baby when you're not in the nursery. Choose between audio-only and video monitors.

6. **Diaper Pail**: An odor-sealing diaper pail helps contain the smell of dirty diapers.

7. **Storage Bins**: Use storage bins or baskets to keep the nursery organized. They're handy for storing toys, blankets, and other items.

8. **Mobile**: A colorful mobile can engage your baby's attention and provide visual stimulation.

9. **Blackout Curtains**: Blackout curtains can help create a dark and peaceful environment for naps and bedtime.

10. **Baby-proofing Supplies**: As your baby grows, you'll need baby-proofing supplies like outlet covers, cabinet locks, and corner protectors to ensure safety.

11. **Nursery Decor**: Add personal touches to the nursery with decor like wall art, curtains, and a rug. Choose soothing colors and themes.

12. **Baby Essentials**: Stock the nursery with baby essentials, including diapers, wipes, clothing, and blankets.

13. **Feeding Supplies**: If you plan to breastfeed or bottle-feed in the nursery, have feeding supplies like a comfortable chair, nursing pillow, and burp cloths.

14. **Sound Machine**: A white noise machine can help create a calming atmosphere for sleep.

Remember to follow safety guidelines for crib placement, ensure all furniture is securely anchored to the wall to prevent tipping, and keep cords out of reach. Setting up a nursery is a wonderful way to prepare for your baby's arrival, and these essentials will help create a safe and comfortable space for your little one.

Decor and Personalization:

Creating a warm and welcoming nursery for your baby involves both decor and personalization. Here are some tips to help you make the nursery a special and comfortable space for your little one:

1. Choose a Theme:
- Select a theme or color scheme for the nursery. Popular themes include animals, nature, classic literature, and more. The theme will guide your decor choices.

2. Wall Art:
- Hang art on the walls that complements the theme. Consider framed prints, canvas paintings, or wall decals featuring animals, characters, or inspirational quotes.

3. Soft Furnishings:
- Use soft furnishings to add comfort and style. This includes curtains, rugs, and plush cushions. Choose fabrics in soothing colors and patterns.

4. Personalized Decor:

- Personalize the nursery with your baby's name or initials. You can find personalized wall art, crib bedding, and more to make the room uniquely theirs.

5. Mobiles and Decorative Elements:

- Hang a mobile above the crib or changing table to provide visual stimulation for your baby. Consider decorative elements like paper lanterns, bunting, or a growth chart.

6. Lighting:

- Install soft, adjustable lighting. A dimmer switch can create a calming atmosphere for nighttime feedings and diaper changes.

7. Storage Solutions:

- Choose furniture that incorporates storage, such as a dresser with drawers or shelves. This helps keep the room organized and clutter-free.

8. Baby's First Library:

- Create a small bookshelf with a selection of baby books. Reading to your baby is a great way to bond, and it's never too early to start.

9. Personal Touches:

- Add personal touches like family photos or handmade decor. These items can help create a sense of familiarity and warmth in the nursery.

10. Safety Considerations:

- When personalizing the nursery, be mindful of safety. Ensure that all decor items are securely attached and out of your baby's reach.

11. Growth Chart:

- Consider adding a growth chart to the wall, which allows you to track your baby's growth over the years.

12. Incorporate Sentimental Items:

- Include sentimental items, such as gifts from friends and family, in the nursery decor. These items can hold special meaning for you and your baby.

-

Remember that the nursery decor should not only be visually appealing but also practical and safe for your baby. Personalization is about creating a space that reflects your family's unique style and welcoming your little one into a loving and comfortable environment.

Safety Precautions:

Safety is a top priority when setting up a nursery for your baby. Here are important safety precautions and babyproofing recommendations to ensure that the nursery is a secure environment:

1. **Crib Safety**:
   - Use a crib that meets current safety standards. Ensure it has no drop sides, and the slats are no more than 2⅜ inches apart.
   - Remove pillows, bumper pads, stuffed animals, and loose bedding from the crib to reduce the risk of suffocation.
2. **Secure Furniture**:
   - Anchor all furniture to the wall to prevent tipping. This includes the crib, dresser, and any tall bookshelves.
3. **Outlet Covers**:
   - Cover electrical outlets with safety plugs or outlet covers to prevent your baby from inserting objects.
4. **Baby Gate**:
   - Install a baby gate to block access to the nursery door if necessary.
5. **Cord Management**:
   - Keep cords from blinds, baby monitors, and other electronics out of your baby's reach and secured to prevent strangulation or tripping hazards.

6. **Radiator and Heater Covers**:
    - Ensure radiators, heaters, and any other potentially hot surfaces are covered to prevent burns.
7. **Toy Safety**:
    - Choose age-appropriate toys that do not have small parts that can be a choking hazard.
8. **Nursery Temperature**:
    - Keep the nursery at a comfortable temperature. Avoid overheating and use a room thermometer to monitor conditions.
9. **Smoke and Carbon Monoxide Detectors**:
    - Ensure there are working smoke and carbon monoxide detectors in the nursery and throughout your home.
10. **Chemical Safety**:
    - Keep cleaning products, medications, and other potentially hazardous chemicals out of reach and in locked cabinets.
11. **Baby-Proofing Latches**:
    - Install latches on drawers and cabinet doors to prevent your baby from accessing hazardous items.
12. **Secure Heavy Items**:

- Ensure heavy or breakable items are secured or moved out of the nursery to prevent accidental injury.

13. **Smoking**:

- Maintain a smoke-free environment to reduce the risk of Sudden Infant Death Syndrome (SIDS).

14. **Safe Sleep Practices**:

- Follow safe sleep guidelines, which recommend placing your baby on their back in a crib with a firm mattress and a fitted sheet, without any additional bedding or sleep positioners.

Regularly inspect the nursery for potential hazards, and as your baby grows and becomes more mobile, adapt the safety measures accordingly. Creating a safe nursery is crucial for your baby's well-being and your peace of mind as you welcome them into your home.

Attending Prenatal Classes

Attending prenatal classes is a valuable and significant aspect of preparing for parenthood. These classes offer numerous benefits for expectant parents, and understanding their importance is crucial. Here are some reasons why prenatal classes are essential:

1. Education and Knowledge:

- Prenatal classes provide comprehensive information about pregnancy, labor and delivery, postpartum care, and newborn care. They cover topics such as stages of labor, pain management options, breastfeeding, and infant CPR. This knowledge empowers expectant parents with the information they need to make informed decisions and feel more confident in their roles as caregivers.

2. Preparation for Labor and Birth:

- Prenatal classes teach various techniques and coping strategies for labor and childbirth. This includes breathing exercises, relaxation techniques, and positions for labor. Understanding the process of labor and what to expect can reduce anxiety and enhance the birth experience.

3. Partner Involvement:

- Prenatal classes often encourage the involvement of partners or support persons. They learn how to provide emotional and physical support during labor and birth, strengthening the bond between partners and enhancing the birthing experience.

4. Social Support:

- Prenatal classes provide an opportunity to connect with other expectant parents. Building a support network of individuals going through similar experiences can be comforting and helpful as you transition into parenthood.

5. Ask Questions and Clarify Doubts:

- Prenatal classes offer a platform for asking questions and addressing concerns. Instructors are there to clarify doubts and provide guidance, ensuring that expectant parents are well-informed.

6. Emotional Preparedness:

- These classes often touch on the emotional aspects of pregnancy, childbirth, and parenting. Expectant parents can learn about postpartum emotional changes and develop strategies for coping with stress and anxiety.

7. Reduce Fear and Anxiety:

- Prenatal classes aim to reduce the fear and anxiety associated with childbirth and parenting. By providing information and practical skills, they help expectant parents feel more at ease and prepared.

8. Early Bonding:

- Learning about infant care, bonding, and newborn behaviors helps expectant parents begin forming an early bond with their baby even before birth.

9. Safety Awareness:

- Prenatal classes often include discussions on safety topics, such as safe sleep practices, car seat installation, and babyproofing, ensuring the safety of the newborn.

10. Postpartum Support: - Some prenatal classes extend their support into the postpartum period, offering guidance on newborn care, breastfeeding, and postpartum self-care.

In summary, prenatal classes offer a comprehensive education and support system for expectant parents, helping them prepare for labor, childbirth, and the early days of parenthood. By attending these classes, expectant parents can build their confidence, reduce anxiety, and gain the knowledge and skills needed to embark on this incredible journey with more confidence and readiness.

Class Options:

Prenatal classes come in various types, each designed to address specific aspects of pregnancy, childbirth, and early parenting. Here are the different class options you can explore:

1. **Childbirth Education Classes**:

- **Overview**: Childbirth education classes focus on preparing expectant parents for labor and delivery. They cover various topics, including stages of labor, pain management options, and breathing techniques.
- **Benefits**: These classes provide knowledge and practical skills to help you navigate the challenges of childbirth with confidence.

2. **Breastfeeding Classes**:

- **Overview**: Breastfeeding classes offer guidance and support for expectant parents planning to breastfeed. They cover topics like latching, milk supply, and common breastfeeding challenges.
- **Benefits**: These classes help parents understand the benefits of breastfeeding and provide the knowledge and techniques for successful breastfeeding.

3. **Parenting Classes**:

- **Overview**: Parenting classes often cover a wide range of topics related to newborn care and early childhood development. They address issues like diapering, feeding, sleep routines, and infant safety.

- **Benefits**: These classes equip expectant parents with essential skills for caring for their newborn, helping them feel more prepared and confident.

4. Lamaze Classes:

- **Overview**: Lamaze classes focus on natural childbirth and pain management techniques. They often include relaxation exercises, breathing techniques, and partner involvement.

- **Benefits**: Lamaze classes are beneficial for those who want to explore natural childbirth options and learn how to work with their bodies during labor.

5. Online Classes:

- **Overview**: Online prenatal classes provide the flexibility of learning from the comfort of your own home. They cover various aspects of pregnancy, childbirth, and parenting.

- **Benefits**: Online classes are accessible and allow you to learn at your own pace. They can be a convenient option for busy expectant parents.

6. Hospital-Based Classes:

- **Overview**: Many hospitals offer their own prenatal classes. These classes are often tailored to the specific services and facilities available at the hospital.
- **Benefits**: Hospital-based classes can provide insight into the birthing process at the hospital where you plan to deliver.

7. Sibling and Family Classes:

- **Overview**: These classes are designed for older siblings and family members to help them understand and adjust to the arrival of a new baby.
- **Benefits**: Sibling and family classes encourage bonding and reduce anxiety for older siblings, preparing them for their new roles.

8. Postpartum and Newborn Care Classes:

- **Overview**: These classes focus on caring for your baby after birth. They cover topics such as diapering, feeding, infant safety, and postpartum recovery for mothers.
- **Benefits**: Postpartum and newborn care classes help parents feel more confident and prepared for the early days of parenthood.

When choosing prenatal classes, consider your specific needs, preferences, and the areas where you feel you would benefit the most. Many expectant parents choose to take a combination of classes to gain a comprehensive understanding of pregnancy, childbirth, and early parenting.

What to Expect:

Prenatal classes are designed to provide expectant parents with valuable information and preparation for pregnancy, childbirth, and early parenting. Here's what you can generally expect during prenatal classes:

1. Topics Covered:
- **Pregnancy Overview**: Classes often begin with an overview of pregnancy, its stages, and what to expect during each trimester.
- **Labor and Birth**: Childbirth education classes will cover the stages of labor, pain management options, and the birthing process. You'll learn about signs of labor, when to go to the hospital or birthing center, and the various stages of labor, including the transition phase and pushing.
- **Breathing Techniques**: Many classes teach different breathing techniques to help manage pain and stress during labor.

- **Pain Management Options**: Prenatal classes typically discuss various pain relief options, including medications and natural methods.

- **Breastfeeding**: Breastfeeding classes provide information on the benefits of breastfeeding, techniques for proper latching, and how to address common breastfeeding challenges.

- **Infant Care**: Parenting classes often cover newborn care topics, including diapering, feeding (breast or bottle), infant safety, and sleep routines.

- **Postpartum Recovery**: Some classes include information on postpartum recovery for mothers, addressing topics like healing after childbirth and managing postpartum emotions.

- **Partner Involvement**: Classes often encourage partner involvement and teach support techniques for labor and delivery.

- **Safety**: Prenatal classes may touch on safety topics such as safe sleep practices, car seat installation, and babyproofing.

2. **Teaching Methods**:

- **Lectures**: Instructors often use lectures to deliver essential information, covering the topics mentioned above in a structured format.

- **Demonstrations**: Instructors may demonstrate various techniques, such as breathing exercises or infant care routines.
- **Hands-On Practice**: Classes may offer hands-on practice opportunities, allowing expectant parents to try out labor positions, diapering, or breastfeeding techniques.
- **Videos**: Videos and visual aids are commonly used to provide real-life examples and illustrations of childbirth and baby care.
- **Discussion and Q&A**: Prenatal classes encourage open discussion and provide opportunities for asking questions and clarifying doubts.
- **Interactive Activities**: Some classes include interactive activities and group discussions to facilitate learning and peer interaction.
- **Support and Community**: Prenatal classes often foster a sense of community among expectant parents, allowing them to connect, share experiences, and build a support network.
- **Homework and Assignments**: Instructors may assign homework or provide reading materials to reinforce what is learned in class.

3. Class Format:

- Classes can vary in duration and frequency. Some classes are held weekly over a few weeks, while others may be condensed into a weekend workshop.
- Classes may be offered in person, online, or as a combination of both to accommodate various learning preferences.

4. Instructor Expertise:

- Prenatal classes are typically led by experienced instructors with expertise in childbirth education, nursing, or related fields. They provide guidance, support, and a wealth of knowledge.

Emotional Preparation:

Emotional preparation is a vital aspect of prenatal classes. These classes are not just about providing practical knowledge; they also focus on helping expectant parents emotionally prepare for the journey of parenthood in several ways:

1. Managing Anxiety and Fears:

- Pregnancy and impending parenthood can bring about anxiety and fears. Prenatal classes address common concerns and provide strategies for managing these emotions. Learning about what to expect during pregnancy, labor, and early parenting can reduce anxiety.

2. Building Confidence:

- Prenatal classes aim to build the confidence of expectant parents. Understanding the birthing process, newborn care, and breastfeeding techniques can instill a sense of preparedness and self-assurance.

3. Emotional Bonding:

- Prenatal classes encourage emotional bonding between partners and with the baby. Learning how to support each other during labor and throughout early parenthood helps strengthen the emotional connection between parents and the baby.

4. Coping Strategies:

- Coping with the physical and emotional challenges of pregnancy, labor, and parenting is discussed in prenatal classes. You'll learn techniques to handle stress, pain, and emotional fluctuations.

5. Partner Involvement:

- Classes often emphasize the importance of partner involvement and provide partners with tools to be emotionally supportive and active participants in the birthing process.

6. Addressing Postpartum Emotions:

- Prenatal classes acknowledge the emotional changes that can occur postpartum. Expectant parents learn about the baby blues, postpartum depression, and how to seek support when needed.

7. Peer Support:

- Connecting with other expectant parents in the class can provide a sense of community and emotional support. Sharing experiences, concerns, and joys can be emotionally enriching.

8. Confidence in Parenting Skills:

- Learning about newborn care, breastfeeding, and safety measures gives expectant parents the confidence that they have the necessary skills to care for their baby.

9. Positive Mindset:

- Prenatal classes foster a positive mindset about childbirth and parenthood. They help expectant parents focus on the joys and rewards of the journey.

10. Communication Skills: - Prenatal classes often include communication exercises to enhance partner communication and ensure a supportive and cohesive parenting team.

In essence, prenatal classes provide not only practical information but also the emotional support and tools necessary for expectant parents to navigate the emotional aspects of pregnancy and parenthood. Emotional preparedness can contribute to a more positive and fulfilling experience throughout the journey of becoming parents.

I hope this information will equip you with the knowledge and guidance you need to create a safe and welcoming nursery for your baby while also preparing you and your partner for the challenges and joys of parenthood through attending prenatal classes. These preparations are crucial for a smooth transition into parenthood and ensuring that you're ready to provide the best care and support for your little one.

Chapter 6

Coping Strategies

In this chapter, we will explore essential coping strategies for expectant fathers as they navigate the emotional challenges of pregnancy, childbirth, and early parenthood. It's natural for dads-to-be to experience a wide range of emotions during this transformative journey, and learning effective coping techniques is vital for maintaining well-being and offering support to their partners.

Breathing Exercises

Breathing exercises are powerful tools for managing stress and anxiety, especially during the emotionally demanding phases of pregnancy and parenthood. These exercises can help you stay calm, centered, and emotionally balanced. Here are some breathing techniques to consider:

1. Deep Belly Breathing:

- Find a comfortable, quiet space to sit or lie down.

- Place one hand on your chest and the other on your abdomen.
- Inhale slowly through your nose, allowing your diaphragm to expand. You should feel the hand on your abdomen rise while the hand on your chest remains relatively still.
- Exhale slowly through your mouth, focusing on a deep, steady breath.
- Repeat this for a few minutes, concentrating on the rise and fall of your abdomen.

2. 4-7-8 Breathing:

- Sit or lie down in a comfortable position.
- Close your eyes and inhale quietly through your nose to a mental count of four.
- Hold your breath for a count of seven.
- Exhale completely through your mouth to a count of eight.
- This cycle can be repeated for a few rounds, calming your nervous system.

3. Box Breathing:

- Visualize a square shape. Inhale for a count of four along one side of the square.
- Hold your breath for a count of four as you move up the square.
- Exhale for a count of four along the next side.
- Hold your breath for a count of four as you complete the square.

- This technique is both calming and grounding.

4. **Alternate Nostril Breathing**:

- Sit comfortably with your spine straight.
- Close your right nostril with your thumb and inhale through your left nostril for a count of four.
- Close your left nostril with your ring finger and release your right nostril, exhaling for a count of four.
- Inhale through the right nostril for a count of four.
- Close the right nostril, release the left, and exhale through the left nostril for a count of four.
- This practice balances and relaxes the nervous system.

5. **Counted Breathing**:

- This technique involves counting breaths to help maintain focus and calm. You can choose a count that feels comfortable, such as inhaling for four counts and exhaling for six counts. The exact count can vary based on your preference and comfort.

6. **Mindful Breathing**:

- Take a moment to pause and simply observe your breath. Pay attention to each inhale and exhale. If your mind starts to wander, gently guide your focus back to your breath. This mindfulness practice can help you stay present and reduce anxiety.

Regularly practicing these breathing exercises can have a profound impact on your emotional well-being and stress management during pregnancy and parenthood. When you feel overwhelmed, take a few moments to center yourself and apply these techniques to regain your emotional balance and offer support to your partner.

Seeking Help When Needed

Recognizing when to seek professional help is a crucial aspect of emotional well-being during the journey of pregnancy and parenthood. It's essential to acknowledge that there may be times when the emotional challenges become overwhelming and that seeking support is a sign of strength, not weakness. Here are some key points to consider:

1. **Signs that Professional Help May Be Needed**:
   - **Persistent Anxiety or Depression**: If you or your partner experience persistent feelings of anxiety, sadness, hopelessness, or other

intense emotions, it may be an indicator of a mental health concern.

- **Difficulty Coping**: If you find it increasingly challenging to cope with stress, anxiety, or the emotional demands of pregnancy and parenthood, professional guidance can be beneficial.

- **Changes in Behavior**: Significant changes in behavior, such as withdrawal from social activities, excessive irritability, or difficulty sleeping, can be signs that professional help is needed.

- **Relationship Strain**: If the emotional challenges are straining your relationship with your partner, seeking couples' therapy or counseling can help address the issues and improve communication.

2. The Importance of Early Intervention:

- Early intervention is often more effective in addressing emotional challenges. Recognizing signs of distress and seeking help promptly can prevent these issues from worsening.

3. How to Seek Help:

- **Talk to a Healthcare Provider**: Your healthcare provider, such as an obstetrician, can be a valuable resource for discussing emotional challenges. They can provide referrals or recommendations for mental health professionals.

- **Contact a Therapist or Counselor**: Licensed therapists or counselors with experience in pregnancy, postpartum, and parenting issues can offer individual or couples therapy.

- **Support Groups**: Joining a support group for expectant or new fathers can provide a sense of community and emotional support. These groups can be in-person or online.

- **Telehealth Services**: Many mental health professionals offer telehealth services, which allow you to access support from the comfort of your own home.

- **Emergency Services**: If you or your partner is in crisis or experiencing thoughts of self-harm or harming others, it's essential to seek immediate emergency assistance.

4. Developing a Plan for Emotional Well-Being:

- It can be helpful to develop a plan for emotional well-being during the pregnancy and postpartum period. This plan may include regular self-care practices, communication strategies with your partner, and a list of support resources.

- Ensure that you and your partner are aware of the plan and the steps to take when emotional challenges arise.

Seeking professional help when needed is an important step in taking care of your emotional well-being as an expectant father. It not only benefits you but also contributes to a healthier and more supportive environment for your partner and the well-being of your family as a whole. Remember that reaching out for help is a courageous and responsible action to take.

Chapter 7

Navigating Challenges

In this chapter, we will explore the common challenges that can arise in a relationship during the journey of pregnancy, childbirth, and early parenthood. It's important to acknowledge that disagreements and conflicts are natural, and finding compromises is key to maintaining a healthy and supportive partnership.

Arguments and Conflicts

As we discussed in chapter 2, communication is very important when certain challenges arise. Remember that disagreements are a normal part of any relationship. They can be opportunities for strengthening your connection and understanding each other better. The key point in effective communication is being open and honest with each other. Express thoughts, feelings, and concerns without judgment. Avoid addressing conflicts in the heat of the moment. Find a suitable time and place for discussion when both partners are calm and receptive. Apologizing when necessary and forgiving each other is a must in resolving conflicts and moving forward. View conflicts as opportunities for personal and relational growth. Use them as a chance to learn more about each other and improve your communication.

Finding Compromises

Finding compromises is a crucial skill in maintaining a harmonious partnership, especially during the journey of pregnancy, childbirth, and early parenthood. Compromises allow you and your partner to manage differences, work together as a team, and find solutions that satisfy both of your needs. Here are some practical tips for negotiation and problem-solving to help you find compromises:

1. Identify Your Priorities:

- Before engaging in a discussion, each partner should identify their priorities and what aspects of the issue are most important to them. Knowing your priorities helps clarify what you're willing to compromise on and what you'd like to maintain.

2. Open and Honest Communication:

- Approach the discussion with open and honest communication. Clearly express your perspective and actively listen to your partner's point of view.

3. Brainstorm Solutions:

- Encourage both partners to brainstorm potential solutions. Even if some ideas seem far-fetched, exploring different options can lead to creative compromises.

4. Be Willing to Give and Take:

- Compromise involves both giving and taking. Be prepared to make concessions and expect your partner to do the same. This balanced approach ensures that both parties contribute to the solution.

5. Avoid Ultimatums:

- Avoid making ultimatums or resorting to a "my way or the highway" attitude. Ultimatums can lead to resentment and damage the relationship.

6. Stay Calm and Patient:

- Keep your emotions in check during negotiations. Sometimes, finding compromises takes time, and it's essential to remain patient and calm throughout the process.

7. Focus on the Bigger Picture:

- Remember that you're working toward a harmonious partnership and a shared future. Keep the bigger picture in mind and consider how the compromise serves the well-being of both partners.

8. Seek Common Ground:

- Look for areas of agreement and shared values. Emphasizing what you have in common can make it easier to find mutually satisfactory compromises.

9. Be Creative:

- Be open to creative solutions that may not fit traditional expectations. Sometimes, thinking outside the box can lead to innovative compromises.

10. Test the Compromise:

- Once a compromise is proposed, test it for a period of time. Assess how well it works for both partners and be willing to make adjustments if necessary.

11. Acknowledge and Appreciate:

- Acknowledge and appreciate your partner's willingness to compromise. Express gratitude and validate their effort to find common ground.

12. Learn from the Process:

- Use the compromise-finding process as an opportunity for growth and learning in your relationship. Understand that finding compromises is a skill that can be developed over time.

Finding compromises is a skill that can strengthen your relationship and improve your ability to work together as a team. By practicing effective negotiation and problem-solving, you can navigate the challenges of pregnancy and early parenthood with mutual respect and understanding.

Chapter 8

Bonding with Baby

In this chapter, we will explore the importance of bonding with your unborn child and supporting your partner's bond with the baby. Establishing a strong emotional connection with your baby during pregnancy is not only beneficial for you but also contributes to the well-being of your growing family.

Connecting with the Unborn Child

Connecting with your unborn child is a beautiful and meaningful experience that can deepen your bond even before birth. Here are various ways to conncct with your baby during pregnancy:

1. Talking to the Baby:
- Have conversations with your baby by gently speaking to your partner's belly. Share your thoughts, hopes, and dreams. Your voice is recognizable to the baby, and talking to them can create a strong emotional connection.

2. Feeling Movements:

- As the pregnancy progresses, you'll likely be able to feel your baby's movements by placing your hand on your partner's belly. Gently stroke or press your hand where you feel movement, and you may even get a response in the form of a kick or a nudge.

3. Playing Music:

- Play soothing or lively music for your baby. Babies can hear sounds from the outside world, and music can be a source of comfort and stimulation for them.

4. Reading Aloud:

- Read books or stories aloud to your partner's belly. This practice not only exposes the baby to language but also creates a calming environment.

5. Attending Prenatal Appointments:

- Accompany your partner to prenatal check-ups and ultrasound appointments. Seeing and hearing the baby's heartbeat and seeing ultrasound images can help you connect with the reality of the pregnancy.

6. Massaging the Belly:

- Gently massage your partner's belly to soothe both her and the baby. You can use a hypoallergenic lotion or oil to make the experience more enjoyable.

7. **Planning Together**:

- Collaborate with your partner on planning for the baby's arrival. Decorating the nursery, choosing baby names, and discussing parenting strategies can be bonding experiences.

8. **Documenting the Journey**:

- Create a pregnancy journal or scrapbook to document the journey. Include ultrasound photos, notes, and your feelings throughout the pregnancy.

9. **Engaging in Prenatal Classes**:

- Attend prenatal classes together to learn about pregnancy, childbirth, and baby care. These classes can provide knowledge and strengthen your bond as you prepare for parenthood.

10. **Sharing in Preparations**:

- Participate in preparing for the baby's arrival by assembling baby furniture, setting up the nursery, and packing the hospital bag.

11. **Offering Emotional Support**:

- Be there for your partner by offering emotional support, understanding her needs, and being patient with her as she navigates the physical and emotional changes of pregnancy.

Connecting with your unborn child not only fosters a stronger emotional bond but also helps you both prepare for the joy and challenges of parenthood. These early connections can pave the way for a nurturing and supportive family environment after the baby's arrival.

Supporting Mom's Bonding

Supporting your partner's bond with the baby during pregnancy is essential for her emotional well-being and for creating a strong family connection. Here are some tips on how to encourage her to connect with the unborn child and provide emotional support during pregnancy:

1. Be an Active Listener:
- Listen attentively when your partner talks about her feelings, experiences, and the baby. Show genuine interest in what she has to say, which can make her feel valued and heard.

2. Encourage Her to Share:
- Encourage your partner to express her thoughts and emotions about the pregnancy. Sometimes, just talking about her experiences can help her connect with the baby.

3. Attend Prenatal Appointments Together:

- Accompany her to prenatal check-ups and ultrasound appointments. Being present during these moments can strengthen her bond with the baby and provide emotional support.

4. Create a Relaxing Environment:

- Create a calm and soothing atmosphere at home. This can help your partner relax and connect with the baby without distractions.

5. Plan Quality Time Together:

- Set aside quality time for the two of you to bond as a couple and share experiences related to the pregnancy. This strengthens your connection and helps you both feel more emotionally connected to the baby.

6. Offer Physical Comfort:

- Offer massages, foot rubs, or physical comfort as needed. These gestures can help reduce stress and create a nurturing environment for bonding.

7. Attend Prenatal Classes Together:

- Participate in prenatal classes together to learn about pregnancy, childbirth, and parenting. These classes can provide valuable knowledge and strengthen your partnership.

8. Share Parenting Resources:

- Share books, articles, or parenting resources that can help her feel more prepared and informed about pregnancy and motherhood.

9. Be Patient and Understanding:

- Pregnancy can bring about emotional and physical challenges. Be patient and understanding when your partner is going through difficult moments.

10. Encourage Self-Care:

- Encourage your partner to engage in self-care activities that help her relax and unwind. A relaxed and happy mom is more likely to bond well with the baby.

11. Share Your Excitement and Enthusiasm:

- Express your excitement about becoming a parent and share your enthusiasm for the baby's arrival. Your positive attitude can be contagious and uplifting.

12. Be Involved in Baby Preparation:

- Participate in preparing for the baby's arrival by setting up the nursery, buying baby essentials, and discussing parenting strategies.

13. Celebrate Milestones Together:

- Celebrate significant milestones in the pregnancy, such as the baby's first kick or hearing the heartbeat. These moments are precious and can strengthen the bond.

14. **Discuss Your Roles as Parents**:

- Have open and honest conversations about your roles as parents. Clarify expectations and support each other in your new responsibilities.

Supporting your partner's bond with the baby is a shared journey that strengthens your relationship and prepares both of you for parenthood. By providing emotional support, understanding, and encouragement, you create a nurturing environment where your partner can connect with the unborn child and feel well-prepared for the joys and challenges of motherhood.

Chapter 9

Building a Support System

In this chapter, we will discuss the importance of building a support system as you prepare for parenthood. Pregnancy, childbirth, and early parenthood can be emotionally and physically demanding, and having a support system in place can make a significant difference.

Involving Family and Friends

Involving family and friends in your journey to parenthood can provide valuable emotional and practical support. Here are some tips on how to effectively involve your loved ones, communicate your needs, and establish boundaries.

1. Communicate Your Needs:
- Open and honest communication is key. Share your needs and expectations with your family and friends. Let them know how they can best support you during this transformative phase.

2. Be Specific:

- When communicating your needs, be specific about what you're looking for. Whether it's help with household chores, emotional support, or childcare assistance, clarity can make it easier for others to provide the right kind of help.

3. Set Realistic Expectations:

- Understand that family and friends may have their own limitations and commitments. While they want to help, be realistic about what they can reasonably offer.

4. Create a Support Network:

- Consider creating a support network of trusted individuals who can provide different types of assistance. For example, one friend may be great at helping with meal prep, while a family member is skilled with childcare.

5. Coordinate Schedules:

- Coordinate schedules with family and friends to ensure that help is available when you need it. This can be especially important during the postpartum period when sleep and rest are crucial.

6. Respect Boundaries:

- While involving family and friends is beneficial, it's equally important to respect their boundaries. Understand that they may have their own lives, responsibilities, and limits.

7. Express Gratitude:

- Show appreciation and gratitude for the support you receive. Small gestures like thank-you notes or a heartfelt conversation can go a long way in maintaining positive relationships.

8. Be Flexible:

- Be flexible and adaptable when receiving help. Things may not always go according to plan, and accepting this can reduce stress and tension.

9. Share Responsibilities:

- Encourage your partner to also share responsibilities when involving family and friends. This ensures that the support system benefits both of you.

10. Establish Privacy Boundaries:

- While you may want support, also establish privacy boundaries. It's important to maintain your family's personal space and intimacy.

11. Seek Emotional Support:

- Sometimes, the emotional support of a trusted friend or family member can be a lifeline. Share your feelings and concerns, and don't hesitate to ask for a listening ear.

12. Set Clear Boundaries with Unwanted Advice:

- Be prepared for well-intentioned but unsolicited advice. Politely set boundaries by saying you'll consider their advice but will make decisions that are best for your family.

Building a support system with family and friends can be a great source of strength during the transformative phase of becoming parents. By communicating effectively, setting clear expectations, and respecting boundaries, you can create a nurturing and supportive environment for your growing family.

Seeking Professional Help

Seeking professional help during the journey to parenthood can be crucial, whether it's for medical concerns, emotional well-being, or parenting advice. Here's guidance on when and how to seek professional assistance:

1. Medical Concerns:
- If you or your partner have any medical concerns during pregnancy, such as unusual symptoms, complications, or discomfort, it's important to consult with a healthcare provider. Don't hesitate to contact your obstetrician, midwife, or family doctor for

guidance. They can address medical issues and provide reassurance.

2. Emotional Well-Being:

- Pregnancy, childbirth, and early parenthood can bring about a range of emotions. If you or your partner experience persistent feelings of anxiety, depression, or overwhelming stress, it's crucial to seek help. Mental health professionals, such as therapists, counselors, or psychiatrists, can provide support and treatment options.

3. Relationship Counseling:

- If you and your partner are facing relationship challenges or conflicts, consider seeking the assistance of a couples' therapist or counselor. They can help you navigate relationship issues and improve communication.

4. Parenting Advice:

- As first-time parents, it's natural to have questions and concerns about parenting. Consult with pediatricians, parenting educators, or attend parenting classes to gain valuable insights and advice.

5. Support Groups:

- Joining support groups for expectant parents or new parents can provide a sense of community and valuable information. These groups can be both in-person and online.

6. Ask for Recommendations:

- When seeking professional help, ask for recommendations from friends, family, or healthcare providers. They can provide insights into trusted professionals and resources.

7. Online Resources:

- Utilize online resources to find professionals, read reviews, and gather information on various services. However, ensure that the sources are reliable and credible.

8. Insurance Coverage:

- Check your insurance coverage to see if professional services, such as counseling or therapy, are included. This can help you choose affordable options.

9. Don't Delay Seeking Help:

- If you or your partner feel the need for professional assistance, don't delay seeking help. Early intervention can lead to more effective solutions and better outcomes.

10. Consult as a Team:

- Make decisions about seeking professional help as a team. Discuss your concerns with your partner and agree on the best course of action together.

Remember that seeking professional help is a sign of strength and responsible parenting. It's an essential step to ensure the well-being of both the expectant mother and father, as well as the growing family. Prioritizing your mental, emotional, and physical health will ultimately benefit your journey to parenthood and the well-being of your child.

Chapter 10

Celebrating the Journey

In this final chapter, we will focus on cherishing the moments of pregnancy and looking forward to parenthood. The journey to becoming parents is filled with emotions, challenges, and transformation. It's essential to celebrate the unique moments and anticipate the joys of parenthood.

Cherishing Pregnancy Moments

Cherishing pregnancy moments is a wonderful way to create lasting memories of this unique and transformative journey. Here are some ways to embrace and appreciate the precious moments of pregnancy:

1. Feel the Baby's Movements:
- Pay close attention to your partner's belly and savor the feeling of the baby's movements. Whether it's the first fluttering kicks or more pronounced jabs, these are moments to be treasured.

2. Create a Pregnancy Journal:

- Start a pregnancy journal to document your thoughts, feelings, and experiences. Include ultrasound images, photos of the growing belly, and any special moments you want to remember.

3. Take Maternity Photos:

- Consider having maternity photoshoots to capture the beauty of your partner's pregnancy. These photos will be a reminder of this precious time.

4. Attend Prenatal Classes:

- Enjoy the learning experience of prenatal classes together. These classes provide an opportunity to bond, gain knowledge, and meet other expectant parents.

5. Plan a Babymoon:

- Take a relaxing babymoon or a short getaway before the baby arrives. It's a special time for just the two of you to celebrate your journey as a couple.

6. Decorate the Nursery:

- Decorating the nursery can be a creative and bonding experience. Choose colors, themes, and decor that resonate with you and your partner.

7. Prepare for Childbirth:

- Attend childbirth preparation classes, discuss birth plans, and explore options for labor and delivery. Preparing for childbirth as a team can strengthen your bond.

8. Take Care of Each Other:

- Focus on self-care and take care of each other during pregnancy. Small gestures of kindness, such as offering massages or preparing favorite meals, can make the experience more memorable.

9. Create a Birth Playlist:

- Create a special playlist of music that you can play during labor and delivery. The songs can be a source of comfort and inspiration.

10. Celebrate Milestones:

- Celebrate important milestones during the pregnancy, such as finding out the baby's gender, completing the nursery, or choosing a name. These moments are worth commemorating.

11. Share Your Excitement:

- Share your excitement with family and friends. Consider hosting a baby shower or gathering to celebrate the upcoming arrival.

12. Reflect and Express Gratitude:

- Take time to reflect on the journey you've been on as expectant parents. Express gratitude for the love, support, and shared experiences.

Cherishing pregnancy moments is about being present in the journey, appreciating each unique experience, and creating memories that you'll treasure as a family. Parenthood is a remarkable adventure, and these moments of pregnancy are the beginning of an extraordinary chapter in your lives.

Looking Forward to Parenthood

Embracing the anticipation of parenthood is a beautiful and exciting part of your journey. Here's how you can look forward to the joys, challenges, and adventures that await you as you step into the world of being mom and dad.

1. Embrace the Joy:
- Parenthood is filled with moments of joy; from the first time you hold your baby to their first smile and milestones. Embrace these moments and let them fill your heart with happiness.

2. Be Prepared for Challenges:
- Parenting comes with its share of challenges. Be mentally prepared for sleepless nights,

diaper changes, and the unpredictability of a newborn. Knowing that challenges are a part of the journey can help you face them with resilience.

3. Stay Open to Learning:

- Parenthood is a continuous learning experience. Stay open to new information and adapt to the changing needs of your child as they grow. Every day is a chance to learn and grow together.

4. Nurture Your Relationship:

- The transition to parenthood can impact your relationship. Make an effort to nurture your connection as a couple by setting aside time for each other and keeping the lines of communication open.

5. Seek Support and Guidance:

- Don't hesitate to seek support from family, friends, or professionals when needed. Parenting can be challenging, and seeking help is a sign of strength.

6. Create Memories:

- Capture the moments of parenthood through photos, videos, and journaling. These memories will be cherished for years to come.

7. Prioritize Self-Care:

- Remember to take care of yourselves. Self-care for both parents is essential to ensure you have the energy and emotional well-being to care for your child.

8. Build a Support System:

- Build a network of support from family, friends, and fellow parents. Having people to share experiences and advice with can be invaluable.

9. Embrace the Adventure:

- Parenthood is an adventure filled with laughter, tears, and moments that will surprise and delight you. Embrace the journey and the unknown and relish the adventure together.

10. Enjoy the Small Moments:

- Parenting is not just about big milestones; it's also about the small, everyday moments of joy. Cherish the simple things, like cuddles, bedtime stories, and shared meals.

11. Celebrate Achievements:

- Celebrate your child's achievements, no matter how small. It could be a first step, a well-behaved day at school, or mastering a new skill.

12. Be Patient with Yourselves:

- Parenting is a learning process, and it's okay to make mistakes. Be patient with yourselves and remember that no one has all the answers.

Parenthood is a remarkable journey that will fill your life with love, laughter, and countless unforgettable moments. While it comes with challenges, it's a beautiful adventure that allows you to watch your child grow, learn, and discover the world. Embrace the excitement and look forward to the incredible experiences that parenthood will bring into your lives.

Your journey as a father-to-be is a remarkable and transformative experience. You've learned about the emotional rollercoaster of pregnancy, the significant role of hormones, and the common mood swing triggers that can affect moms-to-be. You've explored effective communication techniques and coping strategies to navigate the challenges of mood swings and relationship changes during this time.

Understanding the importance of support systems, whether from family, friends, or professionals, is vital for your well-being and that of your partner as you prepare for parenthood. Cherishing pregnancy moments and looking forward to the joys and challenges of parenthood are part of this incredible journey.

As you reflect on your growth as a father-to-be, remember that your love and support are invaluable to your partner and your future child. Embrace the challenges and joys of parenthood with an open heart, a willingness to learn, and a sense of adventure. Your journey is just beginning, and it promises to be one filled with love, laughter, and precious moments that will last a lifetime. Congratulations on this beautiful journey into fatherhood!